MW01077808

Stomach Ulcers Diet

Home Remedies for Curing Sour Stomach, Nausea, and Peptic Ulcers

By

Dr. Junaid Tariq

Stomach Ulcers Diet

Copyright © 2019

All rights reserved. This book or any portion thereof may not be reproduced or used in any manner whatsoever without the express written permission of the publisher except for the use of brief quotations in a book review.

ISBN: 9781698337050

Warning and Disclaimer

Every effort has been made to make this book as accurate as possible. However, no warranty or fitness is implied. The information provided is on an "as-is" basis. The author and the publisher shall have no liability or responsibility to any person or entity with respect to any loss or damages that arise from the information in this book.

MEDICAL DISCLAIMER: All information, content, and material of this book is for informational purposes only and are not intended to serve as a substitute for the consultation, diagnosis, and/or medical treatment of a qualified physician or healthcare provider.

Publisher contact

Skinny Bottle Publishing

books@skinnybottle.com

About the Author

Dr. Junaid Tariq

Backed by 10-years of academic learning and 4 years of research career in medical sciences, I now work as a medical, health and nutrition writer and scientific consultant. My writing is always based on current evidence informed by peer-reviewed journal articles, government and peak health body guidelines, and medical experts, irrespective of the target audience.

My professional focus is on all-natural nutrition and attainable, healthy physiques. I believe that in the modern world when scientists have discovered cures for almost all ailments, there is still no substitute for nature.

Malikjunaidtariq@gmail.com

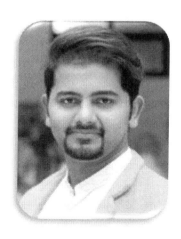

Chapter One

Introduction

Your life is becoming a mess and stress has been your best friend for a while. After spending a few weeks in the blues, you finally get a new job, ace that test, and get the girl. Things are going smoothly until you find yourself struggling with a constant feeling of burning in your chest as if someone is drawing out your soul.

Let's switch to another scenario now.

You often find yourself drained and keep self-medicating on ibuprofen for pain relief until one day your abdomen starts acting funny. You start feeling a nagging pain in the stomach just below the end of your sternum and keep losing weight faster than ever.

Do you find yourself stuck in one of these situations?

Do any of these symptoms seem relatable?

If yes, then I am afraid your stomach might be in a whole lot of trouble. What we are dealing with right now are stomach ulcers.

Do not take stomach ulcers for a minor disease that begins with stomach aches and ends on indigestion.

The disease is capable of troubling you on a whole different level with complications that may even take you straight to your grave (no kidding!). Even if you haven't experienced this situation for yourself, chances are that you would at least have one person in your circle who is struggling with stomach ulcers at a certain point in life.

According to estimates, over 500,000 new cases of stomach ulcers surface on an annual basis within the United States alone, and at a given point, over 5 million people are struggling with this disease.

So, are you sure you haven't heard of stomach ulcers before?

A stomach ulcer is formed when you get a hole or sore in the lining of your stomach. People of any age can get it and both men and women are equally affected by it. Most of the time, it is because of an acquired infection of Helicobacter pylori (H. pylori).

This does not mean that the stress, acid, and spicy foods are not the triggers of this disease.

Why should you worry about stomach ulcers when there are certain prescription medicines to deal with it anyway?

I am not defying the effectiveness of prescription medications in treating stomach ulcers at all. In fact, these medicines might even make you feel a lot better. What these chemical agents are not capable of, is stopping the recurrence. Once you get stomach ulcers, consider yourself stuck in a vicious cycle that keeps bringing these stomach sores back to make your life miserable.

Whether you think you are a victim of stomach ulcers, have recently been diagnosed with this disease, or have been living with it for some time now, this book brings good news!

The diet recommendations proposed to you in this book with a few minor adjustments in the lifestyle will serve as a perfect getaway from stomach ulcers and all the discomfort they have been causing you. In fact, it will serve as a guide that will help you know what foods are suitable, or harmful for your stomach ulcers- it is that simple.

I am strictly NOT in favor of following a strict diet for ulcers from day-to-day making you dread your existence for every single second. Diets are hard to follow and you certainly won't be needing the additional stress induced by "breaking your diet" anyways.

The book is based on the rule that a bland diet might not be effective as a treatment, but at the same time, it is completely harmless. So if following a bland makes you feel better, follow it by all means. There are absolutely no hard and fast rules as different food items affect people differently, even if those foods are highly recommended as a part of the stomach ulcer diet.

So, what are we waiting for? Let's begin the journey towards your transformation!

Chapter Two

Anecdote

September 20, 2014 was an ordinary day for most of us, but not for Diana who woke up only to find herself bleeding profusely. Shocked and frustrated, she knew that something was very wrong. She picked up the phone and called 911 to be taken to the emergency department at once. That was when Diana's life changed, but not for a good reason.

Diana was enjoying her life in Mansfield with her husband, spending quality time with her three children, and being outdoors. But as soon as her stomach pain got worse, Diana got tired easily and her interest in being with others slowly diminished.

She had been visiting the gastroenterologist for a long time. "I endured the sharp pain in my stomach for a really long time and tried to resolve it with antacids," Diana says.

"After having a meal, I would feel a burning sensation in my chest and pain in my upper abdomen. I was unable to get relief from the discomfort of indigestion.

It took a few days and a whole series of medical tests to get her a proper diagnosis. At a tender age of 31, Diana was diagnosed with stomach ulcers. Not one, not two, but a whole bunch of them.

"My frustration stemmed from feeling like that this whole situation could have been prevented with the help of proper medical surveillance".

The mystery was resolved and a list of prescription medications was handed out to Diana but she had other plans. As an attending doctor in the emergency department, I was surprised when I heard her stance.

"I will probably be the last person on Earth who wants to put any sort of chemical medicine into their body," was her response.

Without any further delay, I did what I had to do; a diet transformation. "You can most definitely help yourself feel a lot better sooner and help your body combat this disease by assuring that you're getting the right nutrition," was my agenda to help Diana get out of her misery

I convinced Diana on eating as naturally as she could, particularly focusing on probiotics. Her sheer determination together with a controlled diet worked together to reverse the signs of stomach ulcers and cured her of all the symptoms.

Today, Diana is living a perfectly healthy life free of stomach ulcers without using a single medication. She is enjoying her life and spending quality time with her family and friends.

"Switching to a healthy diet was indeed my turning point," Diana says. *"Diet is a tool, it's not a magic bullet. You have to be willing to induce positive changes in your life and I did. Today, I am completely free of stomach ulcers and the discomfort it brings along. I practically have my whole life back. I have recently started my career in the beauty industry which seemed impossible before this life-changing experience."*

Diana has a great sense of pride that she has healed herself all naturally. If you find yourself in place of Diana and are completely lost, this is the best place for you to be happy, healthy, and hopeful!

Chapter Three

Overview of Stomach Ulcers

Our digestive system is completely dependent on the normal functioning of the stomach. Luckily, this organ has high resistance towards most of the noxious factors such as temperature changes, alcohol, refluxed bile salts, and even the hydrochloric acid that it secretes.

The stomach is an important part of our digestive system.

It plays a pivotal role in the digestion of everything we eat. The mucosa of the inner stomach consists of parietal cells that aid in the digestive processes by the production of gastric juice. Gastric juice, also known as gastric acid, is hydrochloric acid in nature and normally secreted by the stomach cells into the lumen of this organ. The acid is so strong that it makes the pH of the stomach 10 times more acidic as compared to pure lemon juice.

Why do we require gastric acid? It seems tempting to think that you'd be better off without it, but this cannot be farther from the truth.

The gastric juice in your stomach has four important jobs. It initiates proteolysis which is a process by which the proteins are broken down for easy digestion. It activates an enzyme named pepsin which is required for carrying out the normal process of digestion. The hydrochloric acid also aids in chemical signaling so that the food can finally pass from the stomach into the small intestine. At the same time, it also sends signals to the pancreas for releasing its own enzymes. Lastly, the highly acidic pH of the gastric juice also inhibits the growth of bacteria that make their way into the body along with food.

Putting all this together, what is supposed to happen after you have taken your meal? The smell of food is responsible for activating a complex neural pathway that triggers the parietal cells of the stomach to start secreting hydrogen ions. These hydrogen ions form the basis for the gastric juice. As you take a bite of your favorite burger and chew it in your mouth, further stimulation of this pathway occurs, leading to an increase in the production of gastric juice.

By the time you swallow your food and it reaches the stomach cavity, a sufficient amount of gastric acid has already been generated. The pH of your stomach has fallen down to 1 to 2 and the process of digestion pursues. The acid gets mixed with the food bolus and degrades different complex nutrients into simpler forms. Now, the food passes through the pyloric end of the stomach into the first part of your small intestine, also known as the duodenum. The opening of the pyloric valve to let the food pass into the duodenum also requires the presence of proper acid content. Furthermore, this acid is also required for signaling the pancreas which releases its own digestive enzymes into the duodenum to further aid in digestion.

Now that you have developed an understanding regarding the importance of gastric juice in the stomach, a lot of questions might be popping in your head. The most prominent of these questions will be, why does the gastric acid not harm the stomach itself?

The answer to this question is simple- The acid DOES harm your stomach.

In fact, it is totally unbearable for both you and your stomach if the acid production exceeds beyond the limits. It can start burning the layers of the stomach and can even lead to other parts of the body, causing destruction everywhere. But why doesn't this happen? How can the stomach mucosa keep forming HCl without being harmed in the process? And why does the acid in lumen not attack the mucosa?

This is because of the protective barriers or the defense system present in the stomach in different forms. This protective mechanism of the mucosal defense system in the stomach comprises different local as well as neurohormonal factors. This mucosal barrier in the stomach is the special property of this organ which allows the stomach to safely contain all the gastric acid required for normal digestion.

19

The barrier that protects the stomach from the harms of gastric juice consists of three different protective layers. First, there is a compact cell lining comprising epithelial cells. These cells are held together with the help of tight junctions that keep the harsh fluids away which otherwise may damage the stomach mucosal lining. Second, there is a special mucus cover formed by the mucus being secreted by foveolar cells and the surface epithelial cells. The mucus is insoluble and acts like a gel-like coating over the surface of gastric mucosa, protecting it from the corrosive effect of gastric juice. Additionally, it also prevents the auto-digestion of the stomach by pepsin and other materials that you ingest. Lastly, the surface epithelial cells lining the stomach are responsible for the secretion of bicarbonate ions. These bicarbonate ions can neutralize the acidic effect of gastric juice and protect it from damaging the stomach mucosa. Other protective mechanisms that save the stomach from the harmful effects of gastric juices also involve hormonal regulation and the secretion of substances such as prostaglandins.

Now, imagine that due to some reason, the mucosal barrier protecting the gastric mucosa gets weak or completely destroyed? You get a stomach ulcer.

When someone tells you that they suffer from a stomach ulcer, this means that the pepsin and hydrochloric acid build-up in their stomach have destroyed the gastric mucosa. What happens next is that as you eat your meal, the food washes away the acid in your stomach and does not cause any symptoms for the time being. However, when the food is gradually digested and passed on to the intestines, the "raw base: of the ulcer gets exposed to the harmful stomach acid once again which opens it up. This is why you feel the pain and a burning sensation which can sometimes get unbearably strong.

Is stomach ulcers all about bearing the pain your chest and feeling your stomach burn as you gulp down your food?

Research has shown that more than 35 percent of the people who suffer from stomach ulcers tend to develop other complications in addition to the immediate pain. These complications can include a severe perforation of the epithelium lining the gastrointestinal tract and internal bleeding. Stomach ulcers can be pretty painful and can also induce other gastrointestinal systems such as constant bloating, nausea, vomiting, dark tarry stools, and even weight loss. These ulcers may also initiate problems in other systemic organs, particularly in the kidneys and the liver. Stomach ulcers can precipitate chronic kidney disease and may even lead to liver cirrhosis if not managed.

Nevertheless, stomach ulcers do not normally pose a risk of death or an extremely serious illness. Most of the ulcers, up to 90 percent as per some estimates, tend to resolve by dietary modification without any serious medicinal help or surgical procedure.

Chapter Four

The Crux of the Problem

Stomach ulcers have multiple etiologies and can arise from completely unrelated factors. While there can be multiple reasons for stomach ulcers to develop, the most common of them is infection with Helicobacter pylori.

Helicobacter pylori

The Helicobacter pylori (H. pylori) is considered as the main cause of stomach ulcers. The organism was first discovered in the year 1983. Since its discovery, the field of gastroenterology has been revolutionized, particularly in terms of stomach ulcer treatment.

Infections with H. pylori are extremely common and it is possible to get infected with this bacteria without even realizing it. This is because the infection does not manifest itself commonly. This particular species of bacteria reside in the stomach lining and the people belonging to all age groups can be affected by it.

It is considered that one in every three people in their 40's is infected with H. pylori in Australia. Living in the lining of the stomach, it produces chemical and toxins which can sometimes lead to inflammation and irritation. H. pylori is singlehandedly responsible for one-third of the stomach ulcers. It is considered as a contributing factor in three-fifths of the total cases as well. In some people, it can also induce dyspepsia and gastritis.

Stomach ulcers due to H. pylori are particularly disturbing since the infection by this germ can eventually progress to cancers, as per the researchers.

Where does H. pylori come from and how can you acquire it?

The infection by H. pylori is commonly seen in the low-economic areas or the institutionalized people. The modes of transmission of H. pylori are not clear yet. However, it is considered to spread through the sharing of foods, water, and utensils. It can also be acquired by coming in direct contact with the infected vomitus. Some people are naturally more prone to acquiring this infection more than others. The reason for this vulnerability is not known.

Medications

Certain medications are capable of increasing the risk of stomach ulcers by several folds. One such medication includes the category of NSAIDs. NSAIDs stand for nonsteroidal anti-inflammatory drugs. These drugs are commonly used to treat a high temperature, pain, and inflammation in the body. Aspirin, ibuprofen, diclofenac, naproxen are some of the examples of NSAIDs.

NSAIDs are considered as a common cause of stomach ulcers. These drugs have the potential to disturb the mucosal permeability barrier in the stomach. This renders the mucosa vulnerable to injury and eventually, an ulcer develops. As many as 30 percent of the adults relying on NSAIDs for pain management are said to suffer from adverse effects of the gastrointestinal system, stomach ulcers being one of them.

To further understand how NSAIDs can cause ulcers in the stomach, it is important to know how these medicinal agents normally wok. As mentioned before, these medicines are usually taken to reduce pain and treat inflammation, fever, or swelling. There are two enzymes in the human body that secrete chemicals responsible for the development of fever, inflammation, and pain. NSAIDs work by acting on these enzymes and reducing their amounts. Sometimes, these medicines can even completely block the activity of the relevant enzymes just to manage pain or get the body temperature under control.

One of the enzymes that NSAIDs block is responsible for the production of another type of chemical that protects the stomach. This chemical is prostaglandin in nature and its primary responsibility is to maintain the stomach lining and protect it from the harmful effects of stomach juice. As NSAIDs interfere with the normal production of prostaglandins, the safety factor is reduced and the harmful properties of hydrochloric acid override the defense system in the stomach. This ultimately leads to a stomach ulcer.

You are more prone to the development of stomach ulcers in a setting of NSAID use particularly if you have a history of stomach ulcers. Moreover, the risk is higher in female gender and people of older age. Using NSAIDs at a higher dose for the longer duration of time can also increase the risk. Lastly, the use of anticoagulants concomitantly with NSAIDs can also put you at stake for stomach ulcers.

Mental Causes

"ULCERS are no more than fear—tremendous fear of "not being good enough." We fear not being good enough for a parent, we fear not being good enough for a boss. We can't stomach who we are. We rip our guts apart trying to please others. No matter how important our job is, our inner self-esteem is very low. We are afraid they will find out about us"- Louise L. Hay

The role of psychological and mental causes in the development and progression of stomach ulcers can be explained by the narration of a famous incidence. The incident occurred in the early days of the nineteenth century when a man named Alexis Martin shot himself in the abdomen accidentally. Alexis survived the shot but the wound he received was so big that it never completely healed.

A small hole still remained through which his abdominal wall could clearly be visualized. A popular surgeon of that time named William Beaumont decided to observe the abdominal wall of Alexis in order to determine the effect of a man's mood on the process of acid secretion in the stomach. The findings of Beaumont was quite interesting as he observed that the color of the lining changed with a change in emotion. He also observed that the release of acid in the stomach of Martin varied according to the color change. Whenever Martin's faced went red due to anger, the epithelium lining his stomach also changed its color to red.   This observe was manifested in terms of a whole range of moods. All the emotions such as frustration, resentment, anxiety, happiness, and anger were clearly visible on the stomach wall of Martin indicating the connection of the mind to the stomach.

It has been known for ages that different emotions can trigger the development of ulcers. For instance, a feeling of threat allows the brain to trigger acid release in the stomach while reducing the flow of blood at the same time. This ultimately sets the stage for stomach ulcers to form. As discussed above, the presence of H. pylori has also been linked to stomach ulcers by some scientists. However, it is to be noted here that H. pylori is normally found in the stomach of humans. It is similar to the way we have E. coli strains in our intestines and females have a certain type of fungi in their vaginas. The presence of H. pylori in normal circumstances is not harmful to the stomach. This obviously means that there has to be something in the environment that makes people susceptible to the harmful effects of this bacterial species.

Stress and other psychological changes play an important role in this regard.

Scientists today are of the viewpoint that stressful changes in life, such as a feeling of threat or being trapped, can alter the immunity in individuals, leading to the overgrowing of bacteria and making the environment ideal for stomach ulcers. In simpler words, H. pylori can be regarded as the bearer of bad tidings, not essentially the bad news.

The stomach consists of a rich supply of nerves. These extremely sensitive nerves also join with millions of nerve endings in the heart. This is the reason why emotions such as fear, anger, passion, hate, and other feelings can be felt instantly and intensely in this particular area of nerve center. The abdominal area is known as the seat of the subconscious mind and the subconscious mind, in turn, holds a lot of memories from the past. Some of these memories are painful, unjust and bitter. Sometimes, we are instantly reminded of these painful memories and the troubling emotions associated with them in reaction to something that we are doing at the exact moment. It's like one minute you are feeling just fine and the very next minute you have got a knot of shame or fear right in the pit of your stomach.

Rich connections are also seen between the amygdala located in the temporal lobe of your brain and the stomach. These connections permit the intense emotions, such as anger, anxiety, threat, rage, and intimidation, to be felt directly in your stomach. Amygdala is also considered important for the consolidation of memory and can

27

moderate the extent to which a particular traumatic or adverse experience can affect your gastrointestinal system. In animals, this part of the brain is in charge of whether the animals should feel vulnerable or resilient when exposed to stress. A greater feeling of helplessness in the face of aggression, restraint, and the threat will increase the risk of developing ulcers by several folds.

Lifestyle Changes

There is no solid proof whether lifestyle changes can initiate the development of stomach ulcers in individuals. However, some experts are of the view that certain dietary habits such as smoking and drinking can lead to stomach ulcers.

Men who drink more than 2 drinks and women who consume more than 1 drink on a daily basis are more likely to suffer from stomach ulcers. People also believe that spicy food is a key factor for stomach ulcers. While spicy food may not be capable of causing stomach ulcers, such types of food can definitely make the symptoms a lot worse.

Chapter Five

Dietary Modifications for Stomach Ulcers

Now that you are well aware of what stomach ulcers are and how they can attack you, it is time to learn what exactly you can do about it and how can it be done.

Bland diets are one of the most important ways to get your upset stomach back on track. By carefully keeping a track of what you are eating, a bland diet will definitely kill all your stomach miseries and improve your health. I have included a brief introduction to this diet and instructions on how to follow it for your convenience.

Because most of the time, the underlying culprit of the disease is a bacterium, stomach cleanse is usually the best method to overcome it. The process is lengthy and involves different processes. The first part of this process included is adopting a foundational nutrition system. I personally emphasize the importance of this phase as this phase alone may sometimes completely heal your ulcers with dramatic improvements. Phase two of the stomach cleanse restores the normal balance of the microbiome in the digestive system. The stomach cleanse is a gateway for you to know about which nutrients you must take in optimal amounts, for the accurate length of time and in a suitable sequence,

Continue this program at your own pace!

The diet for stomach ulcers will contain a series of suggestions and recommendations for you to follow. I certainly would not want you to be overwhelmed by the information being provided to you. So, it is best to just go through the information once and make notes of the suggestions which can be easily implemented by you. The diet will also guide you to certain food items to completely remove from your diet which must be your prime focus.

Once you have read this book, start off your journey towards a healthy stomach by eliminating all the key foods one by one according to the feasibility. You will be amazed to see the benefits this step might bring you. After the successful elimination of the foods, shift your focus to suitable foods to be used. Bear in mind that it is quite difficult to cater for individual preferences while writing a book.

How quickly will you see improvements?

This is undoubtedly one of the most important and primary questions asked by every person. The genuine answer to this question is, "I don't know". I cannot tell for sure because all of you are unique and have your own set of symptoms and underlying circumstances. Some of you will experience excellent results shortly after eliminating foods. Others will observe gradual improvements as the days pass by and will feel better after a complete stomach cleanse. So, buckle up as your journey towards a healthy stomach begins now!

Chapter Six

What is a Bland Diet?

Traditionally speaking, bland diets have been used to treat a lot of problems related to the stomach such as nausea, vomiting, heartburn, gas, and ulcers. They have also been considered safe to consume right after an intestinal or stomach surgery.

For ulcer patients, these diets have been proposed keeping in mind the fact that the diet must be palatable enough to be eaten. At the same time, it should not stimulate the gastric juices in large amounts as it can further contribute to ulcers. We also tend to feel inclined towards the kind of foods that we seem "comforting" to our upper GI tract. So, we doctors suggest you eating cooked cereals and softly boiled eggs served in breakfast; a simple chicken, fish, or turkey sandwich with decaffeinated coffee for lunch, and dinner consisting of steamed vegetables, pasta, chicken, or maybe some turkey. The fried foods are generally avoided.

Patients usually tend to realize on their own that citrus fruits, such as lemon, orange, or grapefruit, are often poorly tolerated when they have stomach ulcers. They also go for lesser spicy food and completely avoid the ones which are highly seasoned. The whole concept of the bland diet is to provide your digestive tract with soft foods and give it time to recover from all the problems it is currently suffering from, including stomach ulcers.

So, what does this diet consist of?

The following table will give you a general idea of what to expect and how to proceed with a bland diet.

Classification of Food	Suggested Daily Intake	Recommended Foods	What to Limit or Avoid
Milk and other dairy products	2 to 3 servings per day	Fresh, evaporated, or dried milk, yogurt, cream, cottage cheese, and plain cheese	Limit the intake of high-fat dairy
Meat and other protein alternatives	2 servings, each with 2 to 3 oz	Fresh or frozen meat, canned meats (in case	Limit the intake of high-fat meat, fried meat, or meat

	of meat	of salmon and tuna), fish, poultry, eggs, dry beans, seeds, peas, and nuts. Lean or very lean meat must be preferred	dishes with a lot of gravy.
Vegetables	1 to 4 cups (4 to 6 servings)	Vegetables in all forms- fresh, frozen, or canned. Fresh vegetable juice is also recommended	Use minimum amount of au gratin, fried, or cream sauces along with vegetables
Fruits	1 to 2 cups or 2 to 5 servings	Fruits in all forms- fresh, frozen, or canned. Fruit juices are also encouraged	Avocados should be limited
Grains and related products	3 to 10	Prefer enriched or whole-grain bread. Pasta, breakfast cereals, oatmeal, grits, tortillas, popcorn,	Limit the intake of high-fat bread, biscuits, muffins, and other related stuff.

		crackers, cornbread, pretzels, rolls, buns, English muffins, and white/brown rice. It is advised to use at least 3 servings of whole-grain bread on a daily basis	
Nuts, beans, and seeds	4 to 5 every week	All the varieties of nuts, beans, and seeds can be used	
Sweets	1 or less than 1 per day	All types of dessert in a limited amount and portions must be used	Steer clear of high-fat choices

Chapter Seven

Following a Bland Diet

While following a bland diet, all the nutrients are being made available to your body. Only the texture of the regular food items is modified by offering items that follow easy digestion, are low in roughage, and have not passed through excessive seasoning. The focus of the diet is basically on tender foods such as canned fruits, cooked vegetables, cereals, and refined bread. Highly seasoned food, fried food items, caffeinated beverages, pepper, and alcohol might cause stress on your stomach; therefore, they are reduced or completely cut off.

In order to individualize a meal plan according to your suitability, the following guidelines can be followed:

1.   Eat food slowly and chew properly. This is to avoid distention of the stomach which normally occurs when large quantities of food are consumed.

2.   Be sure to eat three times a day. Consume proper meals without any snacks as all food items tend to stimulate the acid output in the stomach.

3.   Use low quantities of salt and a minimal amount of seasoning. Heavy spices such as black pepper, chili pepper, chili powder, and other highly seasoned foods are to be completely avoided.

4.   Milk must be used in a minimal amount as it highly stimulates acid secretion in the stomach.

5.   Dietary fiber can be added to the regular meals as it does not harm the stomach.

6.   Eat whole-grain bread or refined cereals. Steer clear of unprocessed bran, especially in larger amounts.

7.   Observe techniques such as boiling, baking, roasting, broiling, microwaving, stewing, or creaming to cook your food. Avoid frying.

8.   Do not consume tea, coffee, or any other caffeinated beverages because these drinks contain tannins, theobromine, and caffeine.

9.   Avoid taking nonsteroidal anti-inflammatory drugs (NSAIDs) such as aspirin.

10.   Citric juices might not be pleasant, keep their intake to a minimal level.

Now that you are aware of the golden rules of a bland diet, let's move on to the section where we discuss in detail the food items to take or avoid while observing this diet plan

1. Dairy Products

Daily Intake

1-2 servings

What to Eat

- Milk (low fat, whole, or skim)
- Buttermilk
- Milkshakes
- Mild drinks for example pasteurized eggnogs
- Cocoa
- Chocolate milk
- Condensed or evaporated milk
- Yogurt
- Non-fat dry milk solids
- Yogurt with selective fruits
- Soft American cheese
- Mild cheese
- Cottage cheese

What to Avoid

- Strong cheese
- Any food that is generally not tolerated

2. Meat, Poultry, Beans, and Nuts

Daily Intake

2 to 3 servings

What to Eat

- All types of fish (with no bones)
- Very tender chicken
- Lamb
- Beef
- Lean pork
- Veal
- Turkey
- Soft prepared meat alternatives
- Smooth peanut butter
- Tofu
- Finely ground nuts
- Soy cheese
- Eggs

All the meat dishes can be boiled, baked, broiled, microwaved, creamed, stewed, or roasted.

What to Avoid

- Highly seasoned meat
- Fried form of meat

- Cold cuts
- Corned beef
- Sausages
- Ham
- Hot dogs
- Fried eggs
- Chunky peanut butter
- Beans and peas in dry form
- Baked beans

3.   Bread, Pasta, Cereal, and Rice

Daily Intake
6 to 11 servings

What to Eat
- Whole white bread (Refined)
- White bread (enriched)
- Plain rolls
- Crackers (graham or real-time)
- Rye bread (with no seeds)
- Refined cereals (both dried or cooked)
- Hot bread (as per your tolerance)

- Plain spaghetti with no spicy sauce
- Pasta
- Noodles
- Macaroni

What to Avoid

- Course, whole grains
- Highly seasoned crackers with seeds
- Rice or pasta with high seasoning

4. Vegetables

Daily Intake

3 to 5 servings

What to Eat

- White/sweet potato (mashed, creamed, boiled, or baked)
- All canned or cooked vegetables
- Vegetable juices
- Chopped lettuce as per your tolerance

These types of vegetables you decide to choose will highly depend upon your level of tolerance: cabbage, Brussels sprouts, broccoli, cabbage, cauliflower, corn, peas, dried beans, onions, green pepper, sauerkraut, rutabagas, and turnips.

What to Avoid

- Highly seasoned potatoes
- Potato chips
- Fried potatoes
- all vegetables which are not tolerated

Avoid taking fried vegetables. Use raw vegetables with extreme care.

5. Fruits

Daily Intake

2 to 4 servings

What to Take

All types of fruits can be taken in fresh, frozen, or canned forms, as per tolerance

What to Avoid

All fruits with hard skin. Fruits with seeds or uncooked dried fruit must also be prevented.

6. Fats and Oils

Daily Intake

Use sparingly

- Margarine
- Butter
- A low-calorie salad with mild seasoning
- Mayonnaise
- Reduced calorie margarine
- Sour cream
- Oil
- Shortening cream
- Cream cheese
- Cream gravy
- Drained crisp bacon
- Cream sauce

What to Avoid
- All the gravies made using salt pork, meat fats, and fatback
- Highly seasoned salad dressings with seeds

7.   Desserts and Sweets

Daily Intake
Use sparingly

What to Take

- Jelly
- Honey
- Sugar
- Syrups
- Molasses
- Seedless jam
- Non-nutritive sweeteners
- Plain chocolate candies
- Hard candies
- Marshmallows
- Cakes
- Cookies
- Custard
- Sherbet
- Pudding
- Ice cream
- Gelatin dessert

What to Avoid

- Jams with seeds
- Marmalades
- All desserts containing nuts/fruits/coconut
- Fried pastries

- Doughnuts

8. Miscellaneous

Daily Intake
As desired

What to Eat
- Salt
- Herbs
- Mild Spices
- Flavorings
- Gravies and sauces with mild flavors
- Olives
- Soft drinks (free of caffeine)

What to Avoid
- Strong seasonings and condiments like barbecue sauce, chili sauce, and chili pepper
- Black pepper
- Garlic
- Horseradish
- Pickles
- Popcorn
- Coffee

45

- Tea
- Alcoholic drinks
- Caffeinated beverages

You are advised to use lime juice, lemon, vainer, mustard, and catnip with extreme caution.

Sample Menu for a Day

Breakfast
- Half cup of orange juice
- Half cup of scrambled egg
- ¾ cup of cream of wheat
- 1 tsp margarine
- 1 slice toast
- 1 cup of 2 percent milk

Lunch
- ½ cup of white rice
- 3 oz of beef and mushroom gravy (roasted)
- 1/2 cup of carrot coins
- 1 tbsp of French dressing
- 1 cup of iceberg lettuce (shredded)
- 1 slice of bread

- 3 ea of canned pear halves
- 1 tbsp of margarine
- 1 cup of 2 percent milk

Dinner
- 1 cup of macaroni, cheese, and tuna
- Half a cup of peach/banana mix
- ½ cup of string beans
- 1 slice of bread
- 1 sugar cookie
- 1 tbsp of margarine
- 1 cup of 2 percent milk

Bland diet does require you to cut off some food items and limit the others but does not interfere with the total nutrients required by your body. Just to give you a clear idea, the following table has been provided to you. Following the above-mentioned diet plan will provide your body with the following nutrients and minerals in the amounts mentioned beside them:

Riboflavin 3.0 mg	Dietary Fiber 24.2 gm
Vitamin C 95.4 mg	Sodium 2413 mg
Niacin 17.4 mg	Folate 337.9 ug

Phosphorus 1543 mg	Carbohydrate 252.5 gm
Protein 89.0 gm	Fat 81.4 gm
RE Iron 20.7 mg	Calories 2109 kcal
Zinc 25.8 mg	Thiamin 1.7 mg
Calcium 1574 mg	Vitamin A 4327

The amount of sodium that you will be getting from this diet will vary according to the concentration of salt used in daily meals.

Chapter Eight

The Stomach Cleanse- Phase One

Foods to Avoid

Moving towards the dietary modification required for a stomach cleanse and a consequent healing effect on stomach ulcers, the first phase needs to be performed. This phase requires you to get rid of certain foods that might be triggering or aggravating the ulcers within your stomach. Let's discuss these foods one by one in detail.

Gluten

Gluten is a protein commonly found in a lot of food items that you consume on a daily basis. These food items include barley, wheat, and rye. You are likely to be exposed to this particular substance on a daily basis because of a lot of convenience foods, such as pasta,

49

crackers, bread, biscuits, and cakes, are grain-based. It would not wring to consider gluten-containing food items as the mainstay of the western diet, and this is what's causing all the problems. Gluten is also a component of a lot of processed foods as well as different alcohol-based drinks.

What is the Problem?

If you have any kind of digestive systems, including ulcers in the stomach, there is a likelihood of you suffering from gluten intolerance. This is a condition in which gluten can react with your body cells to initiate an immune reaction, ultimately leading to inflammation. Inflammation can adversely affect the process of digestion, not only in the stomach but also in the intestines where it causes the flattening of villi and related disturbances. Continuing to eat gluten in such circumstances can cause serious damage to your digestive system and may even lead to poor absorption of the nutrients.

If you have developed sensitivity to gluten, it is likely that you suffer from certain nutritional deficiencies. For instance, different studies have revealed that gluten sensitivity can lead to a defect in the absorption of vitamin B12 and iron, causing anemia. Other vitamins such as vitamin B1 to B6, lipoic acid, and folic acid can also become depleted. The depletion of these vitamins causes further disturbance in different activities of the body such as detoxification, energy production, and brain functions.

Symptoms of Gluten Sensitivity

It is important for you to know that gluten sensitivity can cause similar symptoms as that of an H. pylori infection. If you are gluten-intolerant, you will suffer from bloating, heartburn, constipation, diarrhea, fatigue, headaches, anxiety, depression, and certain skin conditions. The overlap in the symptoms of both diseases is so strong that people who completely stop taking gluten almost always recover from an H. pylori infection and the consequent ulcers caused by it.

Gluten sensitivity can be called as a hidden plague with different forms. The most severe form of this condition is referred to as Celiac disease. Celiac disease involves a reaction to the gluten that can cause severe pain along with bloodstained stools and diarrhea. However, such patients do not normally suffer from acute digestive symptoms. Instead, they feel more fatigued, depressed, or anxious, suffer from weight fluctuations and anemia. These people may not even get a proper diagnosis of celiac disease unless they have been bone scanned and tested positive for osteoporosis. Gluten sensitivity can be insidious in many ways and can cause hidden damage to the stomach.

It is quite possible that many of your symptoms are occurring because of gluten sensitivity. So, you may benefit a lot by simply removing gluten from your routine meals. Some people tend to experience a great deal of improvement in their symptoms just by controlling their gluten intake. For others, this process takes time as their gut lining requires time to heal properly.

Gluten is Addictive

It may sound easy to completely remove gluten from your diet, but in reality, this can be really challenging. Gluten is found in plenty of foods that you eat on a daily basis. Any food made using rye, wheat, or barley is likely to have gluten in it. This means you will have to say goodbye to breakfast cereals, pizza, biscuits, crackers, lager, beer, and many more of your favorites. Gluten is also used in many processed, canned, or packaged food as a thickener. Do not hassle though as this eBook tends to suggest alternatives that will make you crave less for all the foods you are giving up on.

When you start to avoid gluten, you may experience some cravings. The intensities of these cravings will vary from person to person. In a person who is gluten-sensitive, addictive chemicals are generated by the body when they eat gluten. These chemicals are referred to as Gluteomorphins and they are a lot similar to morphine and heroin, as far as their chemical structures are concerned. Gluteomorphin is also known as gliadorphin and is an opioid peptide that is formed when gliadin, a component of gluten is digested into the body. Gliadin is damaging to the body in some cases such as in autism. It is hypothesized that children who suffer from autism suffer from an abnormal leakage of this compound from their gut. It then passes into the central nervous system and disturbs the brain functions.

If a person dependent on gluten does not take it for a few hours, the levels of Gluteomorphin in the body begin to drop, causing the development of stress and anxiety. This is similar to a withdrawal effect experienced when you suddenly stop taking drugs.

Now that you know about gluten and all the ways it can harm you, how do you know which foods do or do not have it?

Let's simplify it for you!

Good Grains

I personally recommend using the following types of grains. These are considered "good" grains as they are free from harmful molecules of gluten.

- Buckwheat
- Millet
- Rice
- Quinoa
- Amaranth
- Teff
- Corn
- Maize

Foods like bread, pasta, pastries, biscuits, and cakes contain gluten. Similarly, gluten can also be found in different processed foods. A lot of spirits and beers are also made up of gluten. Therefore, it is important for you to find alternatives to these foods. Try using rice cakes, gluten-free bread and pasta, and corn crackers in order to replace these foods. If you absolutely need to use alcohol, drink a very small amount of distilled spirits or wine. Remember never to consume wine on an empty stomach.

Bad Grains

Just to be on the safe side, avoid any food or meal that contains the following items as ingredients:

- Rye
- Wheat
- Wheat flour
- Oats
- Semolina
- Spelt
- Barley
- Couscous
- Beer
- Lager
- Spirits

Do not be confused with ingredients such as 'modified starch' as they are most probably made up of gluten.

The safest and the best way to avoid gluten is by eating a natural diet with whole foods and avoiding any processed item. Oats is an exception on the list of bad grains mentioned above is oats. Oats generally do not contain gluten but most of the time; they are refined in the factories. So, if you really crave for oats, be sure to check if they are processed away from gluten molecules.

Non-Gluten Food Replacements

By far, you have known about the good grains that can be eaten safely and the bad grains which can be problematic. Now, the next question to sort out is what alternatives can be used for the bad grains?

Pasta

You can easily replace your regular pasta with the one which is made up of rice, corn, buckwheat, or millet and is completely free from gluten molecules.

Bread

Gluten-free bread is often available in health food stores. Rice bread is a commonly found alternative in this regard. Additionally, corn crackers and rice can also be used.

Baking

If you are a fan of baking, there are gluten-free alternatives to wheat flour available in the market. Some of these include coconut flour, rice flour, and arrowroot flour. Different recipes can be found on the internet that utilizes these flours.

Spirits and Beers

Cider and wine can be used as an alternative to your alcoholic drinks. However, it is important for you to understand that alcohol is a potential toxin for your body and can disturb different systems such as the liver and the central nervous system.

How much Gluten can You Tolerate?

Research has proven that one-eighth of a teaspoon consisting of wheat flour is sufficient to cause an immune reaction and the consequent inflammation in people who are sensitive to it. Therefore, it is highly recommended to remove all the gluten foods from your everyday diet. Become a food label detective and check labels for everything you buy at the supermarkets to keep yourself healthy and heal the stomach ulcers.

Processed Cow's Milk Foods

If you are suffering from stomach ulcers due to H. pylori infections, you are definitely going to be gluten sensitive as discussed above. However, it is also possible for you to suffer from cow milk intolerance at the same time. Most of the time, any damage caused to your stomach, either by ulcers or any other cause, leads to an increase in the sensitivity of the cells. Sometimes, this also disturbs the cells meant to produce an enzyme named lactase. This enzyme is crucial for you to digest milk and milk-related products. Any kind of damage to these cells leads to a deficiency of lactase. This eventually renders you unable to digest the lactose sugar molecule that is found in cow milk in abundance.

The symptoms produced by lactose intolerance are quite similar to those caused by H. pylori infections or gluten sensitivity. These symptoms include diarrhea, bloating, wind, and abdominal pain. Even if an individual is not sensitive to gluten, he/she can be intolerant to lactose and would not be able to digest products made using cow milk. Some individuals suffering from stomach ulcers react to another substance found in cow milk- casein. Casein is the type of protein often found in cow milk and may cause some people to suffer from the same symptoms as that observed in lactose intolerance.

Once your gastrointestinal lining starts healing due to a gluten-free diet, you may also be able to tolerate cow milk and related products in a period of 60 to 90 days. However, you would need to completely stop taking any product containing cow milk and gluten for a minimum of 60 days. These foods can be introduced again later in life to check if the symptoms return or get worse.

Lactose Intolerance Home Test

In order to adopt a diet in accordance with lactose intolerance, it is crucial to make it clear that you actually have the disease. How can you do it? By taking a simple test at home. This test might not be able to expose each and every case of lactose intolerance but can certainly help you to check whether consumption of cow milk is disturbing your digestive functions.

Start off by completely avoiding milk products for seven days. On the eighth day, wake up and drink a large glass of milk, containing at least 8 to 12 oz of milk, on an empty stomach. Do not eat or drink anything later on, at least for 3 to 4 hours. If you start suffering from symptoms such as diarrhea, gas, bloating, mucus, abdominal discomfort, or any abnormal habits of the bowels, you are suffering from lactose intolerance. In some cases, these symptoms are not immediately evident but appear later during the day, generally within the span of 24 hours.

On the contrary, if the above-mentioned situation does not cause any symptoms in your body, you might not be lactose intolerant. It is important to remember here that while you may be tolerant to lactose, there is a chance for you to suffer from casein allergy which cannot be detected by his test.

Milk is Not the Same Everywhere!

A limited number of products made from cow milk are meant to be used in a raw form. Raw milk can be a promoter of health in many cases. This type of milk is packed with nutrients that can boost the immune system and provide the body with a lot of healthy minerals, vitamins, and friendly bacteria for example Lactobacillus. On the other hand, homogenized and pasteurized milk are not considered to be healthy at all. Unfortunately, most of the dairy products that we use today are pasteurized. The process of pasteurization changes the entire structure of milk proteins and destroys a lot of potentially important nutrients and bacteria in the gut. This can further exacerbate any digestive condition such as stomach ulcers and in order to treat it, such types of milk have to be avoided.

In addition to this, most of the milk produced through commercial farming has a low quality because the cows are fed with low-grade grain foods. Sometimes, these animals are even fed road-kill, further lowering the quality of milk. In many areas of the United States, hormones and antibiotics are fed to livestock, such as cows, which build up in their bodies and can be passed to humans through meat consumption. Cows are meant to eat grass, not any other products such as grain or soy. If you consume any dairy product coming from an unhealthy animal, it is likely for you to be unhealthy as well.

After cutting off cow milk for 60 days, you may try it back to check how it affects you. However, make sure that you use high-quality milk which has not been processed in industries. This is because most of the people who are unable to digest pasteurized milk can easily consume raw dairy products.

Use Sheep and Goat Milk

Another way to reduce the symptoms and severity of digestive issues such as stomach ulcers is by replacing cow milk entirely. Goat milk and sheep milk are perfect alternatives to cow milk for people who cannot withdraw from using milk at all. Alternatively, almond milk or rice milk can also be tried.

Soy

Eating a lot of products containing soy is definitely not going to help you heal stomach ulcers. In your best interest, it is best to cut these products down, and if possible, eliminate from the diet completely.

A few years ago, I was in search of the best solution for those who wished to lose weight. That's when I came to know how soy-based protein shakes which are normally recommended in a weight loss diet must be avoided. I myself used to rely on these shakes a lot some time ago and continuously suffered from digestive problems. Loose stools and flatulence became my best friends. However, it did not take long enough for me to realize that these symptoms were purely because of soy shakes as they resolved the moment I stopped drinking them.

Soy has been called as a healthy food for a few decades. However, it is now considered as a serious problem. A lot of people react to soy in a similar way as they do to gluten. In fact, if you have sensitivity towards gluten and milk, it is likely that you suffer from soy sensitivity as well because soy particles can also cause irritation of the gut lining.

In The Whole Soy Story: Dark Side of America's Favourite Health Food, Dr. Kayla Daniel has mentioned:

"Many studies link soy to malnutrition, digestive distress, immune-system breakdown, thyroid dysfunction, cognitive decline, problems, reproductive disorders and infertility - even cancer and heart disease."

Just like gluten, soy is present in almost two-thirds of all the packaged and processed foods. It is very important to check the food labels of every item and search for the word 'soya' or 'soy'. A lot of products have hidden ingredients containing soy so you might want to look out for these products:

- Soy milk

- Tofu

- Soy infant formula

- Soy protein isolate

- Soyabean oil

- Soy lecithin

- Soy protein concentrate

- Hydrolyzed or texturized vegetable soy

If you are a big fan of soy and cannot think about eliminating it completely, rely on fermented soy products such as natto, miso, tempeh, tamari, and soy sauce. Try to eat these products when you are suffering from soy deficiency in particular.

Sugar

What is the connection of sugar with stomach ulcers? Stomach ulcers caused by H. pylori are particularly affected and aggravated using sugar? How? Because sugar stimulates the overgrowth of yeast. As most of you are trying to rely on antibiotics to treat ulcers, this sets the ground for yeast to grow further. Candida and other fungal infections start to thrive in your body, causing a lot of symptoms. I usually tend to tell my patients that the symptoms they suffer from are probably because of three main factors: H. pylori, food, and secondary infections.

In simpler words, there is something in there that is not supposed to be. If you have additional symptoms of athlete's foot, oral thrush, dandruff, jock itch, burning mouth, brain fog, bread cravings, eczema, and a yellow/white-coated tongue, you are more likely to suffer from a digestive fungal infection that requires immediate attention. Don't worry, as this situation can be controlled to a great extent by just altering your food.

Candida depends upon sugar for growth and minimizing its intake in any form, including the processed carbohydrates such as pasta, bread, cakes, and cookies, can help Candida under control.

Sugar compromises your immunity

Sugar is never good for your body. It can start reducing your body immunity within minutes of consuming it. The presence and proper working of the immune system are necessary in order to overcome stomach ulcers, especially those caused by H. pylori. The complete avoidance is not necessary to stop the infection. Sometimes, the reduction in total sugar intake can also do the trick. However, avoiding sugar and even reducing it can also be extremely difficult.

How can you avoid sugar and all the food items that possibly contain it? Look for the words that end in "ose" on the label. Some of these items include:

- Dextrose
- Maltose
- Lactose
- Sucrose
- High-fructose corn syrup
- Soda drinks
- Soda-pop drinks
- Sports drinks

Other beverages such as lemonade, coke, and other fizzy drinks can contain 8 to 12 teaspoons of sugar in one can. Such drinks can pose a serious threat to your health and may lead to the gradual development of depression, obesity, blood sugar problems, and even skin problems. They are often associated with dental problems and osteoporosis as well.

The role of fruits can also be controversial in this regard. Sugar present in the fruits can also lead to certain problems. You may not realize it but the fruit juices that you buy commercially are so high in sugar that they can be regarded as 'sugar juices'. A glass containing 8 ounces of juice has 8 teaspoons of sugar. Also, these juices are much lesser in terms of fiber as compared to the actual fruit and that's why they cause problems related to the blood sugar levels.

For these reasons, I strictly recommend not consuming any store-bought fruit juices. If you are dependent on juices and cannot think of living without them, try making them yourself at home.

Controlling Your Blood Sugar Levels

While emphasizing the importance of certain foods in the eradication of H. pylori, it is also important to discuss the role of blood sugar. H. pylori infection together with gluten sensitivity can hinder the proper digestion and absorption of food. This causes a disturbance in the blood sugar regulation within the body. Instability in the blood sugar levels and the consequent stress hormone release cause further fluctuations in the levels of blood sugar. This initiates a series of events that ultimately ends up disturbing your immune system.

If you notice your blood sugar levels dropping, it is a sign that your body is producing more amount of cortisol. This cortisol signals the liver to release stored sugar from its warehouse. The body starts relying on cortisol to maintain blood sugar level which ultimately weakens the immune response. This may sound a bit complex, and to make it simple, it is important to regulate your blood sugar levels in order to prevent H. pylori infestation.

The following recommendations might be of value in the regulation of blood sugar:

1.   Make sure that you eat fat and protein during every meal and even while snacking. If you will start relying on carbohydrates only, the blood sugar levels may go up too quickly. This will be followed by a deep drop in the sugar levels, initiating a rollercoaster ride that will make you

stress and disturb your immune system. Proteins and fats can slow the absorption of sugar in your intestines. These can also prevent you from a rollercoaster ride of sugar regulation. So, make sure to consume fats and proteins before eating fruits, grains such as rice, or drinking any vegetable or fruit juice.

2.   Try to eat something every 2 to 3 hours.

3.   Completely avoid foods containing gluten, alcohol, and sugar. This will be a huge step towards balancing your blood sugar and hormones. Moreover, it will also make your immune system healthy and strong.

Fats

Most of the information related to nutrition given to you by the media, the education system, and the physicians are often questionable. This is because this information is biased and depends upon what the food manufacturers want you to believe. In this way, they can sell their highly processed and potentially damaging products and make money.

Coming to the topic, fats are not bad for your health. High-quality fat can, in fact, be regarded as your friend. It is important for you to consume good fats of high quality, especially when you are suffering from gluten sensitivity and stomach ulcers. People who have been suffering from digestive problems for some time are often deficient in certain types of fatty acids. A key step in overcoming stomach ulcers caused by H. pylori is, therefore, to know which fats are good for you and which of them can exacerbate your disease. Some of you will rather be surprised to know that the type of good fats is not quite like what you have imagined.

Good Fats

Following are a few sources which can provide you with good fats:

- Animal fats (from healthy livestock)
- Flax oil (unheated)
- Olive oil
- Coconut cream
- Coconut oil
- Raw dairy (from goats, cows, and sheep)
- Nuts and seeds
- Coconut milk
- Olives
- Avocados (small quantities)
- Egg yolks (whole eggs)

Bad Fats

If consumed in high quantities, the following sources are likely to provide poor-quality fats to your body:

- Avocado oil
- Soy oil
- Sunflower oil

- Peanut oil

- Safflower oil

- Walnut oil

- Cottonseed oil

- Hydrogenated Fats

- Corn oil

- Sesame oil

- Margarine

- Canola oil

- Butter substitutes

- Partially hydrogenated fats

Vegetable oils are commonly believed to be good for health. However, it is not true as such types of oils are quite sensitive to light, oxygen, and heat. These oils also tend to degrade very easily, making it difficult for your body to process them. Oxidation of vegetable oil can, in fact, predispose you to a higher risk of cancer. Therefore, it is extremely important for you to choose the type of vegetable oils you use with extreme care. The following types of oils can be used safely:

- Coconut oil

- Ghee (after avoiding it for 60 days)

- Butter (after avoiding it for 60 days)

- Lard (sourced from organically raised, healthy livestock)

67

You should ideally cook using animal fats and coconut oil. Other vegetable oils, even olive oil, can be damaging to your body, particularly at high temperatures. If you still want to choose olive oil in your food, consider adding it at the end of the cooking so that it is not exposed to high temperatures for a long time.

Using coconut oil is particularly beneficial for your health. It has an additional benefit of possessing antimicrobial properties. Coconuts consist of lauric acid and caprylic acid, both of which can interrupt the process of growth of all yeasts, parasites, and unfriendly bacteria. Monolaurin is also used by a lot of health practitioners to reduce the intensity of diseases caused by H. pylori, including stomach ulcers. The medium fatty chain acids present in the coconut oil are great sources of energy that your body can utilize instantly.

Eating the right kind of fat doesn't make you fat!

There is a lot of misconception regarding fats. Historical evidence has indicated that problems like heart attacks, hypercholesterolemia, and other such conditions did not increase unless we started consuming commercially produced margarine, vegetable oils, and a high volume of sugar. Most of the health problems that occur today are a consequence of high sugar consumption and relying too much on plastic butter-like products and processed oils.

If you are concerned that saturated fats may increase the cholesterol levels in your blood, I insist you go through the following points:

• The primary source of cholesterol in the body is the liver

• Consuming a high amount of sugar is the main cause of high cholesterol in the blood

• Statin drugs are not effective in avoiding heart attacks

• Consumption of cholesterol and fat does not cause an increase in total cholesterol content of the body

When you combine and relate all these points, it will become clear that there is nothing to fear regarding the consumption of healthy oils and fats.

Start being a fat label detective and search the food labels for the kind of fats present in different food items. The following ingredients are to be watched out for in food items:

• Vegetable oil

• Partially hydrogenated vegetable oil

• Hydrogenated vegetable oil

• Peanut oil

• Soy oil

• Sunflower oil

• Safflower oil

69

Chapter Nine

The Stomach Cleanse- Phase Two

Using the Diet Guide

I have tried to make this food diet as easy for you as possible. It is important for you to go through these basic guidelines for further clarifications

1.   The foods written in bold fonts are your primary foods. You are allowed to eat them freely.

2.   The foods written in italics are all secondary foods. These food items must be used occasionally and in smaller amounts. You can also use them as supplementary foods together with the primary ones.

3.   Don't forget to include a primary protein food in every meal. This can include any meat, fish, poultry, or seafood, as per your own liking.

4.   Add secondary foods in your daily meals particularly to give variation, dressings, and flavorings as desired.

5.   If a particular food is not mentioned in the list, do not eat it. You will observe that the list does not contain foods like cakes, pasta, bread, cheese, cow milk, tofu, soy, alcoholic beverages and specific oils such as canola oil. Foods containing gluten and refined sugar have been omitted from the list.

6.   Foods that have a high content of starch, sugar and other carbohydrates are either omitted or placed as secondary foods to help manage the blood sugar.

Meat and Poultry

- Beef
- Buffalo
- Kidney (beef)
- Elk's heart
- Lamb's Liver
- Pork (bacon)
- Pork (chops, ham)
- Rabbit venison
- Chicken (dark and white meat)
- Cornish Hen
- Duck
- Goose

71

- Quail
- Pheasant
- Turkey (dark and white meat)

Fish and Seafood

- Balone
- Salmon
- Cod
- Halibut
- Sardine
- Bass (freshwater)
- Mackerel
- Catfish
- Bass (sea)
- Caviar
- Pompano
- Octopus
- Whitefish
- Mussels
- Rocket Fish
- Clams
- Squid
- Anchovy
- Crab

- Trout
- Scallop
- Tuna
- Crayfish
- Roughy
- Oysters
- Herring
- Grouper
- Lobster
- Perch
- Shark
- Shrimp
- Mahi-mahi
- Snapper
- Swordfish

Legumes

- Aduki Beans
- Black-eyed Peas
- Butter beans
- Broad beans
- Great northern beans
- Chickpeas

- Green beans
- Green peas
- Lentils
- Kidney beans
- Mung beans
- Pink beans
- Navy beans
- White beans
- Pinto beans

Beverages

- Herbal Tea
- Water (Pure or filtered)
- Vegetable Juices
- Black tea
- Caffeinated and decaffeinated coffee
- Fruit juices (freshly squeezed)
- Almond milk
- Rice milk
- Oat milk

Remember not to exceed more than one cup of tea or coffee per day. Prefer taking coffee and tea in the daytime. Avoid processed juices.

Dairy and Eggs

- Feta cheese
- Goat milk
- goat cheese
- goat yogurt
- goat butter
- sheep cheese
- sheep milk
- sheep yogurt
- Egg whites (chicken eggs)
- Egg yolks (chicken eggs)
- Duck eggs (whole)

Where possible, try consuming organic or free-range products.

Vegetables

- Artichoke
- Mushroom (all varieties)
- Asparagus
- Okra
- Aubergine
- Olives (all types)

75

- Avocado
- Onions
- Bamboo Shoots
- Bell peppers
- Shallots
- Beetroot
- Bok Choy '
- Daikon (Asian radish)
- Broccoli
- Fennel
- Reddish
- Brussels Sprout
- Ginger
- Cabbage
- Garlic
- Carrot
- Jerusalem Artichoke
- Cauliflower
- Jicama
- Celery
- Kohlrabi
- Tomato
- Courgette / Zucchini

- Leek
- Water Chestnuts
- Cucumber
- Butternut squash
- Sweetcorn
- Sweet potato
- Turnip
- Swede
- Parsnip
- Potato
- Pepper
- Pumpkin squash

Sea Vegetables

- Agar
- Irish Moss
- Dulse
- Kelp
- Wakame
- Laver

Fruits

- Apples

- Bananas
- Apricots
- Blueberries
- Blackberries
- Boysenberries
- Casaba
- Cherries
- Melon
- Elderberries
- Cranberries
- Coconut
- Cantaloupe
- Grapefruit
- Gooseberries
- Guava
- Grapes
- Honeydew
- Kiwifruit
- Lemons
- Kumquat
- Mango
- Limes
- Nectarines

- Loganberries
- Papaya
- Oranges
- Pears
- Peaches
- Pineapples
- Persimmon
- Plums
- Raspberries
- Pomegranate
- Strawberries
- Rhubarbs
- Watermelons
- Tangerines
- Dates
- Currants
- Raisins
- Prunes
- Figs

Fats and Oils

- Goat butter (without salt)
- Fish oil

- Coconut oil
- Olive oil
- Almond oil
- Borage oil
- Black currant oil
- Hemp oil
- Evening primrose oil
- Sunflower oil
- Sesame oil

Herbs, Seasonings, Spices

- Anise
- Bay leaf
- Basil
- Caraway
- Cayenne
- Cardamom
- Chili powder
- Chervil
- Chive
- Cinnamon
- Cloves
- Coriander

- Curry powder
- Cumin
- Dill
- Fenugreek seeds
- Fennel seed
- Ginger
- Garlic powder
- Horseradish
- Mace
- Mustard
- Marjoram
- Mustard seed
- Oregano
- Nutmeg
- Paprika
- Pepper (ground black)
- Parsley
- Rosemary
- Peppermint
- Salt (unrefined sea salt)
- Saffron
- Sage
- Spearmint

- Savory
- Tarragon
- Turmeric
- Thyme
- Vanilla extract
- Apple cider vinegar
- Rice vinegar
- Wine vinegar
- Balsamic vinegar
- Wasabi
- Dark chocolate
- Carob
- Ketchup
- Hornet
- Molasses
- Mayonnaise
- Brown sugar (unrefined)

Grains

- Buckwheat
- Amarnath
- Oat
- Millet

- Quinoa
- Wild rice
- Brown rice

Chapter Ten

Meal Planning Ideas

Before letting you know how you can plan your meals to heal stomach ulcers, I would like your effort. It is not difficult to change a diet pattern, especially when you have been eating a lot of foods that now you have to avoid. I have listed a few meal plans that are also free of milk, soy, and gluten. At the same time, these meals will also be free of sugar and will consist of the minimum amount of bad fats. I am no chef and the recipes included in the book are just to give an idea about the direction you need to follow. There is always room for improvement and variation according to your style and needs.

Breakfast

It is important for you to consider breakfast as just another meal. Unfortunately, social conditioning has caused us to believe that breakfast comprises of certain foods only. These foods include toasts, cereals, croissants, fruits, and juices. Most of these food items are based on cereals and contain gluten. Also, some of them also require you to use cow's milk with them. The truth is you do not need to use these foods for breakfast only. Your body requires high-quality nutrients and it is completely found to eat any food that is healthy at any time of the day. I hope I don't sound patronizing, but it is important for you to step away from social stereotypes and maintain good health.

Breakfast for Light Appetite

• Boiled eggs with toasted gluten-free bread and an apple

• Corn crackers with 1 to 2 slices of ham, hummus, and an orange

• Rice cakes, soft goat cheese, and a piece of your desired fruit

• Fruit smoothies

Breakfast for a Stronger Appetite

• Small avocado, smoked salmon and olives. You can also make a salad using tomato, lettuce, spinach, and other veggies

• Smoked mackerel fillets with a small avocado, topped with berries

85

• Nitrate-free bacon (Grilled), eggs with cooked yolks and a small glass of any fruit/vegetable juice

• Turkey or chicken salad (both dark and white meat), green lettuce, tomato, celery, parsley, spring onion. For the dressing, you can use olive oil mixed with balsamic or apple cider vinegar.

• Leftovers from last night (this is a clever tactic that helps you eat nutritious food for breakfast)

You can finish your breakfast with an apple or a pear slathered in nut butter such as cashew, peanut, or hazelnut butter. You just have to make sure that the nut butter you use is raw, or made using unroasted nuts. Cooked nuts can damage the delicate oils.

Lunch

• Sliced roast beef mixed with grated goat cheese, peppers, mixed lettuce, mushrooms, onions, with a dressing of apple cider vinegar and olive oil.

• Smoked salmon together with tomatoes, lettuce, olives, and avocados, with a dressing of olive oil and apple cider vinegar. You can also throw in some herbs as an option.

• Celery sticks wrapped in any roast meat slices such as ham. Dip these into soured cream will chives or dills

• Steak with onion, tomato, lettuce, and cucumber

•	Roast chicken with a salad of avocados, tomato, spinach, and olives

•	2 to 3 corn or rice cakes with raw nut butter to any meal.

•	Last night's leftovers

•	Fruit dipped in raw nut butter can be consumed as a dessert

Remember to use apple cider vinegar only when you are not suffering from bloating, burning or stomach pain. Do not consume more than 1 tbsp of vinegar.

Dinner

•	Steak with avocados, eggs, peppers, mushrooms, onions, and olive oil (herb dressing)

•	Chicken thighs with leek, steamed broccoli, kale, and cauliflower

•	Salmon fillets with goat cheese and veggie salad

•	Thai curry or soup with prawns or chicken

•	Familiar meals such as turkey/chicken and chili con carne, vegetable soup, Thai curry dishes, hotspots, stews are perfect choices. Don't forget to add a lot of vegetables

•	Add baked potatoes with a lot of raw goat butter, goat cheese or brown rice with olive oil

Note:

Do not consume starches in large quantities. Small servings must be preferred such as small potato, a handful of carrots, 2-3 new potatoes, or a half cup of rice. Eating too much starchy food together with proteins can be stressful and too much for your digestive system to handle.

Food Quality & Shopping Tips

Buy Organic

Organic food is a bit expensive but highly nutritious and contains a lesser amount of harmful chemicals as compared to commercially grown food. It is also possible for you to get fresh products of extremely high quality at the local farmers market. Because you are going to buy directly from the farmer, the prices are going to be a lot more reasonable as compared to your organic food in supermarkets. Moreover, fresher is always better.

Always be ready to go out of your way to buy in season, locally grown vegetables of the freshest variety instead of buying food at supermarkets. The organic foods available in the supermarkets might be labeled as organic but may not be as nutritious as food grown locally. Search for farmer's market, butchers, or the local cooperatives around your house. Indulge in productive talks with these people to get a feel for how passionate they are about their work and products. You will eventually know that local farmers working on smaller-scale are more concerned about the quality of food they sell in the market. You will rarely find the same passion at a particular supermarket as these markets compete on prices instead of the quality.

Using a good butcher or a farmer's market normally removes a link to the financial retain chain. This makes getting your high-quality food items at less expensive rates. I would also encourage you to search for organic food delivery services. These companies specialize in delivering fresh, organic and whole foods in a lot of areas. So, shop around and find the best one for yourself. If it is absolutely essential for you to shop at a supermarket, stay around the perimeter of the store. The center aisles of these stores are jam-packed with packaged and processed food, but the perimeters are loaded with fresh products.

The food itself must be the sole ingredient and it must not require a label

Don't Get Tricked by Clever Marketing

Terms such as "Natural" or "Organic" written on labels do not essentially mean that a particular food item is healthy. Organic sugar, white flour, and pasteurized milk are not healthy, even if the manufacturers claim it to be grown organically. Remember that usually, the foods which are advertised the most tend to be less healthy. Healthy foods do not need advertisements at all.

Tinned & Frozen Food

Try your best not to buy frozen food. Fresh food is always preferable. This is because freezing usually causes foods to lose their original nutritive value. Home-freezing can, however, be convenient. If you have to choose between tinned or frozen food, always go for the frozen ones since they are better and less harmful to your health.

Meat

If you fail to get your hands on free-range or organic meats, go for leanest cuts. Toxins are primarily stored in the fatty areas of the livestock. When an animal consumes toxins, they are stored in fats because most of them are fat-soluble. When you consume such fats, you are likely to get a dose of these harmful toxins as well.

This rule does not generally apply to the animals that consume a natural diet and live in optimal conditions. This is because such animals are generally healthier and a lot happier. Cows that have spent all their lives in barns and caged chickens in battery farms are to be avoided at all costs.

Poultry & Eggs

A recently published survey by the UK government has shown that organic laying hen farms have markedly reduced levels of Salmonella. This survey has also revealed that 23.4 percent of the farms with caged hens have tested positive for salmonella infections as compared to a small ratio of 4.4 percent in the organic and 6.5 percent in free-range chicken flocks.

Eggs laid by free-range hens have also been shown to have a lesser amount of cholesterol and saturated fats. Such types of eggs have higher levels of omega-3 fatty acids, vitamin Am beta-carotene, and vitamin E. The message I am trying to convey here to go out of your way to prevent battery hens.

Seafood

When you are buying seafood, focus on the smaller species of wild fish. This can include herring, sardines, seabass, and mackerel. Almost all the seafood available in the markets today is contaminated with high levels of mercury. The further up the food chain you want to go, the higher the levels of mercury you are likely to get exposed to. This means that fish species marlin, shark, tuna, and salmon have the highest levels of mercury.

Try your best to avoid farmed fish as they contain the highest levels of toxic metals. For instance, if you notice the flesh of farmed salmon, you will observe that their meat has larger fatty streaks as compared to sockeye salmon or wild Alaskan.

Chapter Eleven

Gluten-Free Recipes

I usually tend to prefer plain foods and simple recipes wherever possible. I have also tried to compile a list of the healthiest recipes. All of them are completely free of cow milk and gluten. These recipes can be cooked in bulk and stored. This will allow you to go through less effort every day while enjoying health diets to cure your stomach ulcers.

Creamy Ham and Bean Stew

What You Require

- 1 tbsp coconut oil
- 1 chopped onion
- Garlic (3 cloves, crushed)

- Diced gammon steaks (450 grams)
- 1 sliced courgette
- 1 chopped red pepper
- 300 ml of chicken stock
- 420 grams of butter beans
- 420 grams cannellini beans
- Black pepper
- Chopped parsley (2 tbsp)
- Goat's yogurt (2 tbsp)

Method

Take a large pan and heat some coconut oil in it. Add garlic and onion and cook it for a few minutes until the onions become soft. Now add the courgette, gammon, and red pepper. Keep frying for a few minutes until the courgette turns brown. Now pour in some chicken stock and let it boil. Turn down the heat and allow it to simmer for 10 minutes. When gammon is thoroughly cooked, add cannellini and butter beans. Season with pepper and salt. Remove it from the stove and finish off with parsley and goat's yogurt.

Moroccan Chicken Stew with Saffron and Apricot

What You Require

- 2 chopped onions

- Coconut oil, 10 grams
- 4 crushed garlic cloves
- A pinch of saffron
- 1 tbsp turmeric
- 1.5 tsp ground coriander
- 1.5 tsp ground cumin
- 1 tsp of black pepper
- 1.5 tsp of paprika
- 8 chicken thighs
- One-fourth tsp of cayenne (do not use it if it irritates your stomach)
- Freshly sneezed lemon juice
- Chicken stock
- Dried apricots, 125 grams
- Chickpeas, 400 grams

Method

Place some oil in a pan and let it stay on medium heat for some time. Add garlic, turmeric, onions, saffron, coriander, pepper, paprika, cayenne, and pepper. Cook all these materials for ten minutes until the onions become soft. Now add chicken, chicken stock, chickpeas, apricots, and lemon juice. Bring the food to a simmering point. Keep cooking gently until the chicken is tender and cooked thoroughly. Serve it with rice.

Pea and Ham Soup

What You Require

- 500 grams of peas (green or yellow)
- 2 chopped onions
- 1.5 tbsp of coconut oil
- 3 celery sticks
- 1 sliced carrot
- 1 kg ham bones/ smoked hock
- A spring of fresh thyme
- One bay leaf
- Lemon juice (as per requirement)

Method

Take a large bowl and place peas in it. Put some water in it and let them soak them for 6 hours. Now heat some oil in the pan and add carrot, onion, and celery. Cook for 6 to 7 minutes. Add hambones, split peas, bay leaves, and thyme together with 2.5 liters of water. Bring it to boil. Reduce the heat for some time and let it simmer, stirring occasionally. Get rid of thyme and bay leaf and removes ham bones. Strop the meat from these bones and chop it. Put this chopped meat back to the soup. Finish off with seasoning using lemon juice and pepper.

Kale, Chorizo and Potato Soup

What You Require

- Chorizo sausages
- Kale, 225 grams with stems removed
- Red potatoes, 675 grams
- Vegetable stock, 1.75 liters
- A pinch of cayenne pepper
- 1 tsp black pepper

Method

Finely chop the kale. Prick the sausages and place them in a pan with enough water to completely cover them. Let them simmer for 15 minutes and cut them into slices. Cook the potatoes using salted water to make them tender. Drain them and mash them to form a paste with some water. Boil the vegetable stock and add kale to it. Also, add chorizo and let it simmer for 5 minutes, now add potatoes and keep simmering for about 20 minutes. Season with peppers.

Mexican Beef Chili

What You Require

- 350 grams of rump steak
- 3 tbsp coconut oil
- 2 chopped onions
- 2 crushed cloves of garlic

- Finely chopped and seeded green chilies
- 2 tbsp mild chili powder
- Tomato puree, 2 tbsp
- 2 bay leaves
- Ground cumin, 1 Tsp
- Beef stock, 900 ml
- 800g canned mixed
- 3 tbsp fresh coriander
- Ground black pepper
- salt

Method

Heat some oil in a large pan and cook the meat on high heat until it turns brown. Remove the meat, lower the flame and add some garlic, onions, and chilies until they become soft. Now add chili powder along with ground cumin and keep cooking fo2 2 minutes. Add back the meat along with tomato puree, bay leaves, and beef stock. Bring the soup to boil and cover the pan. Let it simmer for 45 minutes. Meanwhile, use the potato masher to mash some beans and add to the soup. Add the remaining beans to the soup as it is and keep simmering. Season the soup using coriander.

Irish Country Soup

What You Require

- coconut oil, 15 ml
- 2 quartered onions
- 650 grams of lamb chops cut into small pieces (boneless)
- One liter of water
- Two large potatoes (cut into big chunks)
- Two thickly sliced leeks
- Two carrots
- A spring of fresh thyme
- black pepper to taste
- 2 tbsp of freshly chopped parsley

Method

Heat some oil using a frying pan. Add in some lamb cuts and fry them until they turn brown. Now take them out and add some onions. Now re-add the meat into the pan together leeks. Pour some water and start boiling the solution. Reduce the heat, cover the pan, and let it simmer for 60 minutes. Then, add potatoes, fresh thyme, and carrots in the pan and cook for an additional 40 minutes. Shut the stove and let it stand for five minutes. Don't forget to skim off the fat. Throw in some fresh parsley and serve fresh.

Indian Lamb Soup with Rice and Coconut

What You Require

- Two chopped onions
- Six cloves of crushed garlic
- Root ginger, 5 cm,
- 6 tbsp of olive oil
- Cumin seeds, t tsp
- Black poppy seeds, 2 tbsp
- Ground turmeric, 0.5 tbsp
- Boneless lamb chops, 450 grams (small pieces)
- Rice, 25 grams
- Two pints of chicken or lamb stock
- Lemon juice, 30 ml
- 4 tbsp of coconut milk
- fresh coriander
- Salt and pepper

Method

Use a food processor to process ginger, garlic, onions, and olive oil to form a paste. Set this paste aside. Now take a small frying pan and add cumin, poppy, and coriander seeds and toast it for some time. Use pestle and mortar to grind the seeds. Throw in some ground turmeric. Heat the pan thoroughly and fry the lamb patches on high heat. Remove the lamb and place it aside.

Add garlic, onions, and ginger paste to the pan, cooking it for 2 minutes. Add all ground spices and cook for one minute. Now add cooked meat together with cayenne for seasoning. Finally, add the beef stock and let it boil. Simmer for 30 minutes. Add in the rice and give it 15 more minutes to cook. Lastly, add coconut milk and lemon juice and wait for 2 more minutes. Use bowls to serve.

Spanish Fish Soup with Orange

What You Require

- Hake fillets and trimmings, 1 kg
- 2 pints water
- 2 lemons
- 4 pints water
- 5 garlic cloves
- 2 tbsp coconut oil
- 1 peeled tomato (Chopped)
- 4 potatoes of small size, cut into chunks
- Salt and pepper to taste
- 1 to 2 tbsp of fresh parsley
- 1 tsp of paprika

Method

Cut the fish fillets into small pieces. Lightly salt them and leave them open on a plate. Place the trimmings in a pan and add some water along with the orange peel. Simmer it, skim it, and then cover to cook for 30 minutes. Heat some oil in a deep pan placed on high heat. Crush the garlic cloves and fry them in the pan. After some time, discard it and turn down the heat. Now, fry some onions and add tomato halfway through it. Strain the fish stock and bring it back to boil. Put in some potatoes and cook for five minutes. Add fish and cook for 15 minutes. Season the soup using salt, pepper, and lemon juice. Serve the soup in a bowl.

Chicken and Coconut Soup

What You Require

- 3 tbsp coconut oil
- 40 grams of butter
- 1 freshly chopped onion
- 1 cup of mushrooms
- 2 cloves of chopped garlic
- Fresh root ginger, 2.5cm
- 2 lime leaves
- Half a teaspoon of turmeric
- Coconut milk, 400 ml
- Chicken stock, 475 ml
- Fish sauce, 10 mg
- Spinach, 350 grams
- One lemon stalk
- Chicken thighs, 8 in number

- Spinach, 350 grams

- 2 shallots

- Coconut oil, 30 ml

- Salt and pepper to taste

- 2 tbsp of lemon juice

Method

Heat some oil in the pan and add garlic, onions, and ginger. Let it cook for 4 to 5 minutes. Add the curry paste along with turmeric and cook for further 2 to 3 minutes. Don't forget to stir continuously. Pour in 2/3rd of coconut milk and cook for 5 minutes. Now, add the stock, lemongrass, lime leaves and the chicken. Heat it and simmer for 15 minutes. Remove the chicken thighs and add spinach and the remaining coconut milk. Now process the food using a food processor to smoothen it out. Cut the meat off the chicken bones and make small pieces. Add them in the soup along with lime juice and fish sauce. Gently reheat the soup but take care not to let it boil. At the same time, stir fry some shallots in a separate pan and add them to the soup once they turn golden brown. Use bowls to serve.

Smoked Mackerel and Tomato Soup

What You Require

- Smoked mackerel fillets, 200 grams

- Four tomatoes

- One lemongrass stalk
- Vegetable stock, one liter
- Finely chopped galangal
- Four shallots
- Two cloves of garlic
- Dried chili flakes, 0.5 tbsp
- Thai fish sauce, 1tbsp
- Tamarind juice, 3 tbsp
- A bunch of fresh chives
- Half a teaspoon of brown sugar

Method

Chop the fillets into pieces and separate any stray bones. Take the tomatoes and deseed them after cutting into small pieces. Take the stock and pour it into a large pan. Add some galangal, lemongrass, garlic, and shallots in it. boil it and reduce the heat, simmering it for 15 minutes. Now, add tomatoes, fish, fish sauce, and chili flakes together with tamarind juice and brown sugar. Let it simmer unless heated through.

Serve in bowls

Thai Prawn and Squash Soup

What You Require

- One liter of vegetable stock

- One butternut squash
- Green beans, 90 grams
- Thai fish sauce, 15 ml
- Cooked rice to serve
- Fresh basils (a small bunch)
- Chili paste, one tsp

Method

Peel the butternut squash and cut it into two pieces. Take out its seeds with the help of a spoon and discard them. Now cut the squash to make small cubes. Heat the stock and add chili paste to it. throw in the beans and squash, and let it simmer for 15 minutes. Now add fish sauce, basil, and prawns, simmering for 3 more minutes.

Serve in bowls together with rice.

As I have mentioned a number of times, I know my way around the kitchen, but I am definitely not a chef. These recipes that I have provided are good for your health but might not cater to all the flavors. The reason why I included them is that they are easy to prepare and can be made in large batches. You can alter it according to your needs and taste while keeping in mind to abide by all the rules.

Also, do not add spices if you think they are going to irritate or upset your stomach.

Chapter Twelve

Supermarket Foods to Inhibit H. pylori Ulcers

I have read a lot of studies regarding foods that can kill H. pylori and the resultant infections (even ulcers) caused by it. Although this might not be entirely true, some of these foods still have the capability to reduce the H. pylori disease, if not completely eradicate it.

Based on extensive research, I have put together a list of foods that can either inhibit or eradicate H. pylori in vitro. Eradication of H. pylori is being focused here keeping in mind that more than half of the cases involving stomach ulcers are due to H. pylori.

The food list for H. pylori ulcers includes:

• Berries (raspberries, blueberries, bilberries, elderberries, and strawberries)

- Cranberry
- Garlic
- Tomato
- Olive oil
- Broccoli
- Chili
- Turmeric
- Ginger

Now let's take a look at some of these antimicrobial foods in detail.

Cranberries

Cranberries have been regarded as a fruit that prevents the growth and spread of H. pylori. A study conducted in 2008 on children with H. pylori infections is of particular importance in this regard. The study found that children who utilized cranberry juice experienced a reduction in the H. pylori infections by 16.9 percent as compared to only 1.5 percent in the control group. In 2007, a few Israeli researchers reported that cranberry juices also have an ability to enhance the potential benefits of antibiotics in treating H. pylori infections. The results of a trial involving 177 patients suffering from H. pylori infection, posted in the journal named Molecular Nutrition & Food Research indicated that drinking cranberry juice during the entire length of a weeklong antibiotic course and even after it can speed up the bacterial eradication up to 10 percent.

Broccoli & Broccoli Sprouts

Broccoli consists of a component known as sulforaphane. The sprouts of broccoli are specifically high in this component. In 2002, a research team led by Dr. Jed Fahey indicated that sulforaphane can inhibit the growth of H. pylori in the infected mice.

It is also important to note here that other cruciferous vegetables such as cauliflower, cabbage, and Brussels sprouts also consist of this very agent and may also be used as superfoods for the eradication and prevention of H. pylori and the consequent ulcers. Vitamin U, which is not a vitamin as opposed to its name, is found in cabbage and cabbage juice and is particularly famous for its properties to heal stomach ulcers.

Olive Oil

Olive oil is frequently used as a base for preparing home-based salad dressings. I strictly recommend that this oil must not be cooked at high temperatures as it loses its stability and might become denatured. If you do not like adding olive oil to your sauces, consider sprinkling it at the end of your food preparation. In other words, do not expose this oil to high temperatures to save yourself from health troubles later.

A study conducted by the scientists belonging to de la Grasa, a Spanish institute, indicated that certain chemicals known as polyphenols present in olive oil possess antibacterial activity against 8 different strains of H. pylori. Out of these 8 strains, 3 are currently resistant to antibiotic treatment as well. Olive oil is also considered as a health-promoting oil, so it is also good to be consumed on a daily basis regardless of its activity against H. pylori.

Garlic

The active ingredient in garlic is allicin, a potent antibacterial agent. Throwing in half a clove of fresh garlic while making a fruit or vegetable juice at home, or simply consuming it with a meal can help your body get rid of all the unwanted bacteria in the digestive system. You can also eat it in raw form. However, you need to be careful while consuming garlic as too much of it can cause bad breath and body odor. Moreover, an excess of everything is bad so, don't overdo it. one clove of garlic is sufficient per day. Don't forget to check the necessary precautions if you are already taking blood-thinning medicines.

Although garlic has been shown to possess antimicrobial properties, its role in killing H. pylori is slightly controversial as some studies have failed to monitor any improvement in the infected patients. But why not give it a try?

Green Tea

A recent experimental trial has also shown that certain compounds present in the composition of green tea can successfully inhibit an infection caused by H. pylori in vitro. Green tea has also been found to reduce stomach inflammation in mice.

Cayenne Pepper

Cayenne does not specifically kill H. pylori infections directly. However, this particular food item is said to enhance the levels of the IgA antibody secreted from the mucosa of the digestive tract. In case you are not aware, IgA antibody is considered as your first line of defense against different foreign invaders including H. pylori, yeasts, and parasites. The levels of this antibody tend to drop, especially if you are suffering from digestive infections, gluten sensitivity, or stress.

Cayenne can help to increase the levels of the IgA antibody by increasing the amount of blood flowing to the mucosa of the stomach. In this way, it strengthens the body's natural defense system against all bacterial infections. You can consider adding half a teaspoon of cayenne to water or a juice mix. However, take care not to consume too much of it as it is a type of spice and overconsumption can irritate your stomach.

Chapter Thirteen

The Stomach Cleanse- Phase Three

The stomach cleanse protocol is a program in which you utilize nutritional supplements that have been scientifically proven to have negative effects on H. pylori infections and ulcers.

When I suffered from ulcers caused by H. pylori, my symptoms included stomach pain, heartburn, belching, nausea in the morning, and constipation. All of these symptoms were reduced to a great extent three days after I started stomach cleanse and were completely gone by the end of the fourth week. I am not claiming that this program will work best for all of you with the same rate of discovery. However, it can benefit the majority of you.

The best thing about a stomach cleanse is that you can completely rely on it for the reduction of your H. pylori-induced ulcers. Moreover, it can also be used in combination with the antibiotics of the famous triple-therapy treatment. It is completely compatible with medicines and can be safely consumed during your regular antibiotic course. It is my personal belief that the nutritionists and other naturally oriented practitioners must work together with the medical physicians towards recovery.

Timing of the Stomach Cleanse

I highly recommend you run a stomach cleanse program after following the diet plan for H. pylori mentioned in the earlier chapters. You should be following it for 8 to 12 weeks, or 60 to 90 days before you start this course. Why is that important? Because this nutrition program will lay a base for the final phase of stomach cleanse to work. It will also allow your stomach to manage any inflammation and heal itself as far as possible. In case any symptoms fail to disappear during the diet program, phase three of the stomach cleanse is going to take care of it.

I would like to remind it again that the diet meant for H. pylori might not be able to treat your stomach ulcers completely. The purpose of this diet is just to improve your overall health, reduce inflammation and stress, and to bring your hormones into a perfect state of balance. Only then will your body be able to experience the stomach cleanse properly and work synergistically with it to heal completely.

If you do not follow the Dietary recommendations, the stomach cleanse will not work because of the following reasons:

- Continuing to eat cow milk, gluten, and soy products would not reduce inflammation in your stomach. The cortisol levels will not normalize and continue to disrupt your immune system

- Your immune system will be compromised if you keep eating unchecked

What are the best supplements for stomach cleanse?

Berberine

Berberine is a component of different herbs such as barberry, goldenseal, and Oregan grape. It has been indicated to possess broad-spectrum activity against different bacteria and microbes. In vitro studies have demonstrated that berberine can stop H. pylori but might not be able to completely eradicate it.

Deglycyrrhizinated Liquorice Root (DGL)

DGL is an established agent for ulcers as it consists of mucosal healing properties. It can coat the intestinal lining and provide soothing effects that can ultimately heal the inflamed tissues and ulcers. Research has suggested that certain flavonoids present in the licorice have strong antimicrobial activity against H. pylori strains. These flavonoids also work against the strains of H. pylori resistant to antibiotics such as amoxicillin and clarithromycin, the primary antibiotics against bacterial invasion used in triple therapy. Some types of licorice are believed to raise the blood pressure, but because GDL has fairly low levels of glycyrrhizin, it is safe to take it even if you are a patient with high blood pressure.

Manuka Honey

Manuka honey takes its origin in New Zealand. It is frequently promoted as a food item that can effectively kill H. pylori along with all of its complications. While this might be the case, it is important to keep in mind that honey is basically sugar. You know that certain species of yeast such as Candida need sugar to thrive and you also know about the connection of H. pylori infections and secondary fungal infections as well. For this reason, I will not force you to use Manuka honey as a part of your stomach cleanse as there are far better alternatives present in the market.

This does not mean that you should rule manuka honey out completely as it might be able to benefit you on an individual basis.

Mastic Gum

Mastic gum consists of bismuth in its composition. Bismuth-containing medications are often recommended in a quadruple therapy together with antibiotics. If you use bismuth, it is likely to turn your stools black. It is not recommended to use this supplement for more than 60 days in a row. Mastic gum can, however, must be used in safe limits as doctors all around the world are continuously arguing about its useful effects in treating digestive problems including ulcers in the stomach.

Siberian Pine Nut Oil

Siberian pine nut oil has been receiving mixed reviews regarding its usefulness in the treatment of H. pylori infections. This particular agent is not backed up by any scientific trial that proves its efficacy. However, a lot of cases have emerged proving that it has anti-bacterial properties.

Sulforaphane

Sulforaphane is a naturally existing chemical, commonly found in cruciferous vegetables such as cabbage, broccoli, and Brussels sprouts. A large number of studies have indicated its capacity to stop H. pylori infections. Eating cruciferous vegetables such as broccoli sprouts will make sure that your body gets sufficient quantities of sulforaphane.

Additionally, sulforaphane is also available commercially in the form of capsule and supplement form.

Vitamin C

A number of studies have suggested the role of vitamin C in killing H. pylori infection. It has been concluded in different pieces of literature that vitamin C therapy for infection against H. pylori infection might be clinically relevant but more research is required in order to determine the dosage and the duration of therapy.

Even if vitamin C fails to eradicate H. pylori completely, it is still worth taking as studies have proven how H. pylori infections can significantly reduce the levels of vitamin C.

This is particularly because of the oxidative and inflammatory stress exerted by this organism in the stomach. Vitamin C is also an essential nutrient that speeds up the gut healing and can be used as a part of stomach cleanse.

Vitamin U

Vitamin U is also known as MSM and is commonly found in raw forms of cabbage. As opposed to its name, vitamin U is not a vitamin in real. Cabbage juice has been examined extensively in the Eastern European countries for its role in healing the eroded and damaged mucosa of the digestive tract. The studies have revealed that this agent is of special importance in healing damaged tissue and for this very reason, it can be used in stomach cleanse to treat ulcers.

Zinc-L-Carnosine

Zinc-L-Carnosine does not possess any antimicrobial properties as such. However, it is an excellent choice for repairing damage caused to the stomach. It is also useful to heal ulcers in the stomach. Taken together with other agents possessing anti-microbial properties, Zinc-L-Carnosine can be a perfect choice for a stomach cleanse.

Can stomach cleanse be used alongside triple therapy?

My answer to this question is, why not? Stomach cleanse comprises all-natural ingredients that you are normally taking in the form of foods. That is why it is completely safe to continue stomach cleanse alongside your normal treatment plan. If you are planning to use a commercial supplement as a part of stomach cleanse, it would be better to consult a physician first before pairing it up with triple therapy.

Can children use the stomach cleanse?

Stomach cleanse programs can be used in children to overcome H. pylori infections. Everything recommended as a part of this program is natural, therefore, cannot harm them. The dose can be reduced as per requirements. Otherwise, it is a completely safe program for children as well as adults

Conclusion

Stomach ulcers are nasty and can make your life miserable within days, but with the right kind of diet and proper meal plans, all of your miseries can go away. Always remember that eating well is a form of self-respect and it has the power to create health in all areas of life. By following the dietary guidelines given in the book, you will not only be treating stomach ulcers but also saving yourself from a lot of other health hazards that you might have encountered in the future.

Eat well and stay well!

Junaid Tariq

One last thing!

I want to give you a **one-in-two-hundred chance** to win a **$200.00 Amazon Gift card** as a thank-you for reading this book.

All I ask is that you give me some feedback, so I can improve this or my next book :)

Your opinion is *super valuable* to me. It will only take a minute of your time to let me know what you like and what you didn't like about this book. The hardest part is deciding how to spend the two hundred dollars! Just follow this link.

http://reviewers.win/stomachulcers

Made in the USA
Las Vegas, NV
18 April 2023

70763971R00066